MW00876696

Hiatal Hernia Syndrome

A Beginner's 3-Step Plan to Managing Hiatal Hernia Syndrome Through Diet, With Sample Recipes and a Meal Plan

mf

copyright © 2022 Patrick Marshwell

All rights reserved No part of this book may be reproduced, or stored in a retrieval system, or transmitted in any form or by any means, electronic, mechanical, photocopying, recording, or otherwise, without express written permission of the publisher.

Disclaimer

By reading this disclaimer, you are accepting the terms of the disclaimer in full. If you disagree with this disclaimer, please do not read the guide.

All of the content within this guide is provided for informational and educational purposes only, and should not be accepted as independent medical or other professional advice. The author is not a doctor, physician, nurse, mental health provider, or registered nutritionist/dietician. Therefore, using and reading this guide does not establish any form of a physician-patient relationship.

Always consult with a physician or another qualified health provider with any issues or questions you might have regarding any sort of medical condition. Do not ever disregard any qualified professional medical advice or delay seeking that advice because of anything you have read in this guide. The information in this guide is not intended to be any sort of medical advice and should not be used in lieu of any medical advice by a licensed and qualified medical professional.

The information in this guide has been compiled from a variety of known sources. However, the author cannot attest to or guarantee the accuracy of each source and thus should not be held liable for any errors or omissions.

You acknowledge that the publisher of this guide will not be held liable for any loss or damage of any kind incurred as a result of this guide or the reliance on any information provided within this guide. You acknowledge and agree that you assume all risk and responsibility for any action you undertake in response to the information in this guide.

Using this guide does not guarantee any particular result (e.g., weight loss or a cure). By reading this guide, you acknowledge that there are no guarantees to any specific outcome or results you can expect.

All product names, diet plans, or names used in this guide are for identification purposes only and are the property of their respective owners. The use of these names does not imply endorsement. All other trademarks cited herein are the property of their respective owners.

Where applicable, this guide is not intended to be a substitute for the original work of this diet plan and is, at most, a supplement to the original work for this diet plan and never a direct substitute. This guide is a personal expression of the facts of that diet plan.

Where applicable, persons shown in the cover images are stock photography models and the publisher has obtained the rights to use the images through license agreements with third-party stock image companies.

Table of Contents

Introduction

If you're grappling with the discomfort of a hiatal hernia, you know it's far from a picnic. This ailment, characterized by a portion of the stomach protruding through a gap in the diaphragm, can lead to symptoms that are quite troublesome. But there's good news: your diet can play a significant role in managing your symptoms, and perhaps even in supporting your body's ability to heal.

A hiatal hernia can make you feel like you're on a roller coaster of discomfort, but it doesn't have to dictate your life. You're not alone in this; many have trodden this path before, searching for solace in their daily meals while avoiding the dreaded flare-ups.

The Hiatal Hernia Diet isn't about strict limitations or taking away all the foods you love. It's about understanding which foods can help soothe your symptoms and which might trigger them. It's a thoughtful approach to eating - one that emphasizes balance, variety, and moderation, geared towards enhancing your comfort and well-being.

With a few strategic choices, you can create a friendly environment for your digestive system. This means selecting foods that are less likely to cause reflux, one of the primary symptoms of a hiatal hernia. From the texture of what you eat to the timing of your meals, each aspect of your diet contributes to your overall symptom management.

In this guide, we will talk about the following;

- What is Hiatal Hernia Syndrome?
- Symptoms, Causes, Diagnosis, and Treatments of Hiatal Hernia
- Natural Methods to Manage Hiatal Hernia Syndrome
- 5 Step-by-Step Plan to Manage Hiatal Hernia Syndrome
- The Hiatal Hernia Diet
- Principles, Benefits, and Disadvantages of Hiatal Hernia Diet
- Foods to Eat and to Avoid
- Sample Meal Plan and Recipes

You'll also uncover how small adjustments to your eating habits can have a positive impact on your quality of life. Envision enjoying a quiet night without the nagging heartburn, or savoring a favorite meal without the aftermath of pain and discomfort. It's about reclaiming the joy of eating and adapting to your body's new needs.

As you continue reading, you'll be equipped with knowledge that empowers you to take charge of your hiatal hernia through diet. Remember, small steps can lead to significant improvements in how you feel day-to-day. With this guide, you're on your way to crafting a personalized eating plan that aligns with your health goals, brings comfort, and restores a sense of normalcy to your life at the table.

Let's delve deeper and explore how the Hiatal Hernia Diet can become a cornerstone of your strategy for managing your symptoms and enhancing your overall wellness.

What Is Hiatal Hernia Syndrome?

Hiatal hernia syndrome is a medical condition where a portion of the stomach pushes through an opening in the diaphragm, known as the hiatus, and protrudes into the chest cavity. Under normal circumstances, the stomach resides beneath the diaphragm.

The term "*hiatal*" refers to the hiatus—the hole in the diaphragm that separates the chest and abdominal cavities. A hernia happens when a weak spot in the body allows an organ or other soft tissue to push through it.

This condition can lead to various symptoms and complications. It's often associated with gastroesophageal reflux disease (GERD) and difficulty swallowing. In severe cases, it can result in ulcers or Barrett's esophagus.

There are two primary types of hiatal hernias: sliding and paraesophageal hernias.

Sliding hernias

This type occurs when a part of the stomach pushes up through the esophageal hiatus. They represent about 95% of all hiatal hernia cases. Often, they do not cause symptoms and thus, do not necessitate treatment.

Paraesophageal hernias

These are less common but potentially more problematic. The stomach pushes through next to the esophagus, which can lead to the stomach being trapped and its blood supply being cut off, causing serious issues.

Hiatal hernias are quite common, affecting approximately 20% of the population. The condition is more prevalent in women than in men and tends to occur more frequently as individuals age.

Symptoms of Hiatal Hernia

A hiatal hernia is a condition where part of the stomach pushes through the diaphragm into the chest cavity. The following are the most common symptoms of hiatal hernias:

- *Heartburn*: The individual experiences a burning sensation in their chest, typically after eating. This symptom tends to worsen when they lean over or lie down.
- *Chest pain or epigastric pain*: They feel discomfort or pain in the area between the neck and the abdomen.
- *Trouble swallowing*: Eating becomes difficult as they struggle to swallow food or liquids.

- *Belching*: They frequently burp, which can be uncomfortable.
- *Upset stomach or nausea*: They often feel sick to their stomach, which can affect their appetite and overall well-being.
- *Regurgitation of food or liquids into the mouth*: Partially digested food or bitter-tasting stomach acid occasionally flows back into the mouth.
- *Acid reflux*: They experience a backflow of stomach acid into the esophagus, causing a sour taste in the mouth and potentially leading to other complications if not managed.
- *The feeling of fullness soon after eating*: They feel unusually full shortly after starting to eat.

It's important to note that some individuals with a hiatal hernia may not experience any noticeable symptoms. If someone is experiencing any of these symptoms, it's crucial for them to seek medical advice.

Causes and Risk Factors

The exact causes of hiatal hernia syndrome are not fully understood, but it is thought to be caused by a combination of factors like age, anatomy, diet, and lifestyle.

- *Age*: Hiatal hernias are more common in older adults, which may be due to the weakening of the diaphragm and other abdominal muscles with age.
- *Anatomy*: Some people are born with a larger hiatus, which can make them more likely to develop a hiatal hernia.
- *Diet*: Eating large meals or lying down immediately after eating can increase the risk of hiatal hernia syndrome.
- *Lifestyle*: Obesity, smoking, and pregnancy can all contribute to the development of hiatal hernias.
- *Obesity*: Excess weight puts pressure on the stomach and can lead to a hiatal hernia.
- *Smoking*: Smoking can contribute to a hiatal hernia by weakening the lower esophageal sphincter muscle.
- *Pregnancy*: The increased abdominal pressure during pregnancy can cause or worsen a hiatal hernia.

Hiatal hernias are also more common in people with certain medical conditions like GERD, diabetes, and connective tissue disorders.

Diagnosis

Hiatal hernia syndrome is often diagnosed based on symptoms and a physical examination. Your doctor will ask about your medical history and perform a physical exam to look for signs of a hiatal hernia.

In some cases, your doctor may also order tests to confirm the diagnosis. These can include:

Upper GI series

An Upper GI series, also known as a barium swallow, is a radiographic examination that involves taking X-ray images of the upper digestive system. Patients drink a barium solution, a chalky, dense liquid, which coats the lining of the esophagus, stomach, and small intestine.

This contrast material makes any abnormalities visible on X-rays, allowing doctors to diagnose conditions such as strictures, ulcers, hiatal hernias, tumors, or other anomalies.

Esophageal manometry

Esophageal manometry is a diagnostic procedure designed to assess the pressure and muscle contractions within the esophagus. During the test, a thin, flexible catheter is inserted through the patient's nose and gently guided down the throat into the esophagus. The catheter has pressure sensors that detect the strength and coordination of esophageal muscles as the patient swallows.

This is particularly critical for evaluating the function of the lower esophageal sphincter (LES), which acts as a valve between the esophagus and stomach. By measuring these pressures, doctors can diagnose conditions like achalasia or other motility disorders that may cause symptoms such as difficulty swallowing, chest pain, or reflux.

pH monitoring

pH monitoring is a diagnostic test that records the level of acidity in the esophagus over a period of 24 to 48 hours. A thin sensor, often attached to a strip of tape, is positioned above the lower esophageal sphincter to continuously measure esophageal pH levels. This sensor transmits data wirelessly to a portable recorder carried by the patient.

Accurate pH measurements help doctors diagnose and manage conditions like gastroesophageal reflux disease (GERD) by identifying abnormal acid exposure in the esophagus, correlating acid reflux episodes with symptoms, and assessing the efficacy of acid-suppressing medications.

Endoscopy

Endoscopy, specifically esophagogastroduodenoscopy (EGD), is a minimally invasive diagnostic procedure that allows physicians to visually examine the esophagus, stomach, and beginning of the small intestine. A slender, flexible tube equipped with a camera and light, called an endoscope, is gently inserted through the patient's mouth and guided down the throat.

As the camera transmits real-time images to a monitor, the doctor can spot inflammation, ulcers, tumors, or other abnormalities. The procedure is instrumental in diagnosing various gastrointestinal conditions, obtaining biopsies, and sometimes treating identified problems.

Treatment

There are several treatment options available for hiatal hernia syndrome. The best treatment option for you will depend on the severity of your symptoms. It is best to talk to your doctor about the best treatment option for you.

- *Medications*: Many different medications can be used to treat hiatal hernia syndrome. These include antacids, H2 blockers, and proton pump inhibitors.
- *Antacids*: Antacids work by neutralizing stomach acid. They are available over the counter and can provide relief from mild symptoms.

- **H2 blockers**: H2 blockers work by reducing the amount of acid produced by the stomach. They are available over the counter and by prescription.
- **Proton pump inhibitors**: Proton pump inhibitors work by reducing the amount of acid produced by the stomach. They are available by prescription.
- **Surgery**: In some cases, surgery may be necessary to treat hiatal hernia syndrome. Surgery is typically only recommended for people with severe symptoms who do not respond to other treatments.

Hiatal hernia surgery is typically performed through a small incision in the abdomen. The surgeon will then repair the hernia and tighten the lower esophageal sphincter muscle.

Natural Methods to Manage Hiatal Hernia Syndrome

Several natural methods can be used to manage hiatal hernia syndrome. These include:

Exercise

Exercise can help to reduce the symptoms of hiatal hernia syndrome. Exercise can help to strengthen the muscles around the stomach and esophagus. This can help to prevent acid reflux. Some exercises that may be helpful include:

- **Yoga**: Yoga can help to relax the muscles around the stomach and esophagus.

- *Pilates*: Pilates can help to strengthen the muscles around the stomach and esophagus.

Avoid trigger foods

Certain foods can trigger the symptoms of hiatal hernia syndrome. These include fatty foods, spicy foods, caffeine, and alcohol. It is best to avoid these trigger foods. The next chapter will get into more detail about trigger foods.

Eat smaller meals

Eating smaller meals can help to reduce the symptoms of hiatal hernia syndrome. When you eat a large meal, it can cause the stomach to distend. This can put pressure on the lower esophageal sphincter muscle and lead to acid reflux.

Elevate your head

Elevating your head can help to reduce the symptoms of hiatal hernia syndrome. When you sleep, elevate your head by placing pillows under your head and shoulders. This will help to keep stomach acid from rising into the esophagus. You should elevate your head for at least 30 minutes after eating.

Avoid tight clothing

Tight clothing can put pressure on the stomach and lead to acid reflux. It is best to avoid tight clothing, especially around the waist. Some examples of tight clothing include:

- Tight pants

- Tight belts
- Tight waistbands
- Tight shirts
- Tight dresses

Wear loose-fitting clothing

Wearing loose-fitting clothing can help to reduce the symptoms of hiatal hernia syndrome. Loose-fitting clothing will not put pressure on the stomach. This can help to prevent acid reflux. Some examples of loose-fitting clothing include:

- Loose pants
- Loose skirts
- Loose shirts
- Dresses with a loose waist

Sleep on your left side

Sleeping on your left side can help to reduce the symptoms of hiatal hernia syndrome. When you sleep on your right side, it can put pressure on the stomach and lead to acid reflux. Sleeping on your left side will help to keep the stomach below the esophagus.

A 5-Step Guide to Manage Hiatal Hernia Syndrome

Deciding to manage your syndrome not only by taking medications recommended by your doctors is a huge step, especially if the lifestyle you're used to is different from the lifestyle recommendations described in the previous chapter.

It's understandable if you choose not to rush it because doing so may do more harm than good. What's best is to prepare your mind and body to adjust to these changes you'll be starting for your overall well-being.

One of the best ways is to plan what exactly it is you want to focus on. For example, if you want to make sure that diet and exercise are two of the things you want to stick to doing for a long time, then make sure you incorporate ways on how you can stick to following a diet program and an exercise routine for the long term.

Here below is a 5-step guide to get you started on this journey:

Step 1: Consult with Your Healthcare Provider

Commencing any natural management techniques for hiatal hernia pain necessitates a prior conversation with a healthcare provider. This crucial step ensures that you avoid potentially detrimental practices and instead adopt safe, effective strategies. A provider, knowledgeable about your health history and the intricacies of hiatal hernias, can offer insights into non-invasive management options.

Dietary modifications might seem straightforward, but they can inadvertently cause nutrient imbalances or interact with existing medical conditions. Expert guidance is indispensable to craft a comprehensive and balanced dietary plan that doesn't just target symptom relief but also supports overall health and well-being.

Dietary Adjustments

An essential component of managing hiatal hernia pain naturally involves revisiting your eating habits. Since many trigger foods—such as spicy dishes, fatty foods, and caffeine—are prevalent in daily consumption, eliminating these items abruptly can be daunting and impractical. A gradual approach is often more sustainable and less disruptive.

Collaborate with a doctor or a dietitian to identify which foods exacerbate your hernia symptoms and learn how to phase them out or replace them with healthier alternatives. These modifications should be carefully calibrated to maintain a varied and nutritionally rich diet that meets all of your body's requirements.

Medication Consultation

While there exist over-the-counter medications that purport to alleviate symptoms related to hiatal hernias, such as antacids or acid reducers, it's prudent to seek a physician's recommendation before taking them.

Your doctor can advise on the most appropriate medication based on the severity of your symptoms, your overall health, and any other medications you are taking, thus avoiding unwanted side effects or drug interactions. This personalized approach to medication ensures both safety and efficacy in managing your condition.

Lifestyle Modifications

Non-medical factors can significantly influence the frequency and severity of hiatal hernia symptoms. Discuss with your healthcare provider the aspects of your daily routine that may need to be adjusted, such as your choice of clothing (tight belts or waistbands can increase abdominal pressure) and your sleeping posture (elevating the head of the bed may reduce nocturnal reflux).

These lifestyle modifications can substantially improve your quality of life when tailored to your specific condition and habits. Solicit your provider's expertise for creative solutions if standard recommendations do not resonate with you or seem difficult to implement.

Ongoing Medical Support

Lastly, managing a chronic condition like a hiatal hernia is an ongoing process that benefits from continuous medical oversight. Keep your healthcare provider informed about the natural methods you are incorporating into your management plan, and establish a schedule for regular follow-up appointments.

These visits are opportune times to assess the effectiveness of your approaches, address any new or persisting symptoms, and make necessary adjustments to your regimen. This ongoing dialogue ensures that your self-management strategies are not only effective but also evolve in concert with your lifestyle and health status, guaranteeing a comprehensive approach to your condition.

Step 2: Stick to a healthy diet and keep a food diary

Learning to curate a proper diet will be useful in this journey. Start by learning to understand the types of food that will both be beneficial and harmful for you. Then, from there, try to find different recipes that will appeal to you and provide you with the necessary nourishment to properly meet your daily needs.

Slow diet transition

Ideally, not overdoing it when you just started is a smart move. Incorporate your healthier meals slowly but surely, say, start with eating one healthy meal every two days. Then, in the following week, level it up by assigning three alternating all-healthy meal days, then do it for five days. After that, if you think you've adjusted well to this type of diet, then do it for an entire week and do your best to keep up with it.

The transition doesn't have to be done weekly. You can do it bi-weekly or perhaps every 10 days. Adjust this according to your preference, just make sure that you will do your best to achieve your goal of fully eating healthy in the long run. Here's a weekly meal plan you can either follow or modify according to your means or preference.

	Breakfast	Lunch	Dinner
Day 1	Fresh Asparagus Salad	Sun Crust Turkey Cuts	Korean-Style Cauliflower
Day 2	Cauliflower and Mushroom Bake	Macrobiotic Bowl Medley	Baked Turkey Wings
Day 3	Spinach, Feta, and Tomato Omelet	Arugula and Mushroom Salad	Rice Noodles with Chicken

Day 4	Squash and Spinach Medley	Rice Noodles with Chicken	Fruit Salad with Zesty Vinaigrette
Day 5	Grapefruit and Spinach Smoothie	Orange-Walnut Salad	Blackberry Cobbler
Day 6	Low-Cholesterol Apple-Cinnamon Granola Breakfast	Korean-Style Cauliflower	Rice Noodles with Chicken
Day 7	Orange-Walnut Salad	Baked Turkey Wings	Rice Noodles with Chicken

Food diary

As you start following a stricter diet that will be very helpful to your condition, try to keep a food diary where you'll take note of how the meals are, what you feel after eating, or if there are things you want to modify. While it may seem tedious at first, you'll find that doing so will be beneficial for you for a long time. The food diary will also be useful on your corresponding visits to the doctor.

You should be able to keep watch on the food that is healthier and is not prone to triggering acid reflux. You can also keep an eye on when you have trouble digesting or are experiencing other stomach-related symptoms.

You can also keep a food tracking app like MyFitness App, MyPlate Calorie App, and FatSecret to name a few.

Some of these apps also include features that keep track of your exercises or other activities. Make sure that you include information about your symptoms and triggers and when they occur.

Keeping a food diary is a good thing to do especially at the beginning of your diet. As previously mentioned, one of the recommended ways to manage the symptoms is to decrease the amount of food you consume per meal. It's not ideal to just do this drastically as it may be even harmful to you. Taking note of the gradual changes in your meal serving in your diary will help you slowly keep track of and eventually maintain this change.

Here's a sample food diary template you can copy or modify:

Day and Time of Meal	Food (Ingredients)	Serving	Notes/Remarks
Monday Lunch	Spinach, Feta, and Tomato Omelet	1	Experienced stomach ache
Monday Dinner	Turkey Wings	1	Had to adjust my meal but I felt full
Tuesday Breakfast	Apple-Cinnamon Granola Breakfast	1	One serving is enough
Tuesday Lunch	Asparagus Salad	1	Besto to change one ingredient with another

After one week, review your food diary and look for patterns. Are there certain foods that seem to trigger your symptoms? If so, avoid these foods.

Starting a diet is always stressful and challenging because it forces you to change not only your usual menu but also your eating habits. Keeping a diary where you can write down your struggles or keep notes of your ups and downs during the diet journey can somehow lessen the burden of these major changes.

Step 3: Be Active and Slowly Adapt to Healthy Changes

Incorporate gentle physical activity into your daily routine to support your hiatal hernia diet. Start with low-impact exercises such as walking, swimming, or yoga, which can help strengthen the diaphragm and abdominal muscles without putting too much pressure on your hernia.

Exercise with Caution

Listen to Your Body: Begin with short durations of activity and gradually increase as you become more comfortable. If any exercise causes pain or discomfort, stop immediately and consider alternative movements.

- *Avoid Heavy Lifting*: Steer clear of lifting heavy objects or performing strenuous activities that can increase intra-abdominal pressure and potentially worsen your condition.

- *Stay Upright Post-Meals*: After eating, try to stay upright for at least an hour. This position helps prevent stomach contents from pushing against the hernia, reducing the risk of reflux.

Adapt Your Diet Gradually

- *Introduce New Foods Slowly*: As you eliminate trigger foods, introduce new, healthier options one at a time. This will make it easier for you to identify any foods that may still be problematic.
- *Adjust Meal Sizes and Frequency*: If switching to smaller, more frequent meals is challenging, make the transition slowly. Gradually reduce the size of your main meals while adding small snacks between them.
- *Stay Hydrated*: Drink plenty of water throughout the day, but avoid drinking large amounts during meals, as this can add volume to your stomach and pressure to your hernia.

Embrace Lifestyle Changes for Long-Term Success

- *Prioritize Sleep*: Ensure you get sufficient quality sleep each night. Consider elevating the head of your bed slightly to prevent acid reflux during the night.
- *Manage Stress*: Chronic stress can exacerbate hiatal hernia symptoms, so find stress-reduction techniques

that work for you, such as deep breathing exercises, meditation, or engaging in hobbies.

- *Monitor Your Progress*: Keep track of your dietary changes, physical activity, and hiatal hernia symptoms. This log will help you notice patterns and the impact of your lifestyle changes on your health.

By being active and making gradual, healthy changes to your diet and lifestyle, you'll not only manage your hiatal hernia symptoms but also improve your overall well-being. Remember that consistency is key, and making these changes a permanent part of your life will provide the best long-term relief.

Step 4: Optimize Your Eating Environment

Creating a conducive eating environment can significantly impact the management of your hiatal hernia symptoms. The setting in which you consume your meals plays a crucial role in digestion and can either alleviate or aggravate your condition.

Create a Relaxing Mealtime Atmosphere

- *Minimize Stress*: Eat in a calm and quiet space to reduce stress levels, which can impact the severity of acid reflux. Avoid eating while working, driving, or watching television.

- *Set the Table*: Make mealtime special by setting the table. This encourages you to sit down and focus on your food, aiding in mindful eating.

Ensure Proper Posture While Eating

- *Sit Upright*: Maintain good posture during meals. Sit up straight with your shoulders back to avoid compressing your stomach, which can push stomach contents into the esophagus.
- *Take Breaks*: If sitting for a full meal is uncomfortable, consider standing or taking a short walk between courses to aid digestion and alleviate pressure.

Adjust Timing for Meals and Snacks

- *Regular Meal Times*: Establish and stick to consistent meal times. This regularity can help your digestive system function more effectively and prevent overeating.
- *Last Meal Timing*: Have your last meal or snack well before bedtime to give your body time to digest food properly, reducing the risk of nighttime acid reflux.

By focusing on a peaceful and proper eating environment, you can help soothe your hiatal hernia symptoms and improve your overall digestive health. Remember that your eating habits are just as important as what you eat when it comes to managing this condition.

Step 5: Regularly Evaluate and Adjust Your Approach

The final step in managing your hiatal hernia through lifestyle changes involves regular self-evaluation and flexibility to adjust your approach as needed. It's important to acknowledge that managing a hiatal hernia is an ongoing process that may require tweaks to your strategy over time.

Monitor Your Symptoms and Triggers

When making lifestyle changes to manage your hiatal hernia, it's essential to keep track of any symptoms you experience and what may have triggered them. This will help you identify patterns and adjust your habits accordingly.

Keep a Symptom Diary

Maintaining a detailed symptom diary is a cornerstone of managing a hiatal hernia. By meticulously recording each instance of discomfort alongside your meals, stress levels, and exercise habits, you create a valuable database. This log enables you to discern which foods or activities may exacerbate your symptoms.

Over time, patterns emerge from this data, offering insights into the complex interplay between your lifestyle choices and your hiatal hernia symptoms. Equipped with this knowledge, you can make informed decisions to avoid potential triggers and maintain a better quality of life.

Review and Reflect

Dedicating time each week to review your symptom diary is crucial for the effective management of your hiatal hernia. This reflective practice allows you to analyze recorded patterns and understand the impact of your lifestyle modifications.

You can identify what has been successful in mitigating your symptoms and what has not, enabling a proactive approach in tailoring your daily habits. Consistent reflection enhances your awareness of your condition and empowers you to make adjustments that align closely with your body's needs, fostering an environment conducive to healing and comfort.

Stay Informed and Adapt

By staying informed about your hiatal hernia and keeping up with the latest research, you can make educated decisions when it comes to managing your symptoms. Make use of reputable sources such as medical journals and healthcare professionals to expand your knowledge and understanding of this condition.

Stay Updated on Research

To effectively manage a hiatal hernia, it is vital to stay educated on the evolving landscape of medical knowledge. Advances in research may bring forward new recommendations or treatments that could be beneficial.

By subscribing to health newsletters, following relevant medical journals, and engaging with online patient communities, you can remain at the forefront of current findings. This proactive approach ensures that your management strategies are supported by the most recent evidence and best practices in digestive health care.

Be Open to Change

Flexibility in managing your hiatal hernia symptoms is key. As you track your triggers and responses, be prepared to modify your diet and lifestyle based on what you learn. If certain foods or exercises consistently lead to discomfort, consider exploring new alternatives that align better with your condition.

Engaging with healthcare providers, nutritionists, and even support groups can offer fresh perspectives and solutions tailored to your needs. Embrace change as an opportunity for improvement and actively seek out adjustments that can enhance your well-being.

Consult with Healthcare Professionals

It's essential to maintain consistent communication with your healthcare provider through regular check-ups. During these visits, your doctor can closely monitor the progression of your hiatal hernia and evaluate the effectiveness of your current management plan.

These sessions are also the perfect opportunity for you to receive personalized medical advice and have any new symptoms assessed. Your provider may suggest adjustments to your treatment based on the latest medical insights, ensuring that your approach remains both effective and safe.

Emphasize Progress Over Perfection

When managing a chronic condition like a hiatal hernia, it's important to remember that progress is not linear. There will be good days and bad days, and that's completely normal.

Celebrate Small Victories

When managing a hiatal hernia, it's important to recognize the journey is made up of small steps. Every positive change, no matter its size, is a victory worth celebrating. These milestones, such as a day free of discomfort or successfully avoiding a known trigger, are significant achievements that contribute to your overall progress. Celebrating these moments can boost your morale, reinforce your commitment to your health, and provide motivation to continue making beneficial choices every day.

Be Patient and Persistent

Adapting to the lifestyle changes necessary for managing a hiatal hernia requires patience and persistence. It's a long-term commitment, and improvements in symptoms might unfold gradually. Understand that it's normal for progress to ebb and flow. Maintaining a patient and persistent mindset helps you to stay focused on your goals, despite any setbacks.

Over time, with consistent effort, you are likely to notice a cumulative impact on your well-being and a more controlled management of your symptoms.

By continuously evaluating and adjusting your approach to managing your hiatal hernia, you can maintain control over your symptoms and enhance your quality of life. Stay proactive about your health, and remember that with the right strategies, you can live comfortably despite a hiatal hernia.

The Hiatal Hernia Diet

A Hiatal Hernia diet refers to a specific eating plan designed to help manage the symptoms associated with a hiatal hernia. A hiatal hernia occurs when part of the stomach pushes up through the diaphragm into the chest cavity, which can cause discomfort and various digestive issues.

The primary goal of this diet is to minimize these symptoms and prevent further irritation or exacerbation of the condition. In the next section, we will discuss the Principles, Benefits, and disadvantages of the hiatal hernia diet.

Principles of Hiatal Hernia Diet

The principles of the Hiatal Hernia diet revolve around minimizing symptoms such as acid reflux, heartburn, and discomfort that are associated with a hiatal hernia. Here are the core principles:

- *Eat Smaller, More Frequent Meals*: This helps prevent the stomach from becoming too full, which can put pressure on the LES (lower esophageal sphincter), potentially causing or exacerbating acid reflux.

- *Limit Acidic and Spicy Foods*: Foods with high acidity or spice can irritate the esophagus and stomach lining, worsening symptoms.
- *Reduce Intake of Trigger Foods*: Certain foods like chocolate, caffeine, fatty foods, carbonated beverages, and alcohol can relax the LES, making reflux more likely.
- *Avoid Eating Before Bedtime*: Lying down with a full stomach can encourage acid to flow back into the esophagus. It's generally recommended to stop eating at least 3 hours before lying down.
- *Maintain a Healthy Weight*: Excess weight, especially around the abdomen, can increase abdominal pressure and cause more frequent acid reflux.
- *Eat Slowly and Chew Food Thoroughly*: Eating in a rushed manner can lead to swallowing air, which can increase gastric pressure and worsen hiatal hernia symptoms.
- *Stay Upright After Meals*: Gravity can help keep stomach contents down, so it's advised to stay upright for a while after eating.
- *Wear Loose Clothing*: Tight clothing around the midsection can squeeze the stomach and force food up against the LES, promoting reflux.

- *Consider Food Preparation*: How food is prepared can also impact symptoms. Grilled, baked, steamed, or poached dishes are often better than fried or fatty ones.
- *Stay Hydrated with Non-Irritating Beverages*: Drinking water and other non-irritating beverages can help in digestion and maintaining overall health without increasing the risk of reflux.

These principles are meant to guide dietary choices to manage hiatal hernia symptoms effectively. It is always advised to consult with a healthcare professional for personalized dietary advice.

Benefits of the Hiatal Hernia Diet

The Hiatal Hernia diet offers several benefits aimed at managing symptoms and improving the quality of life for individuals with this condition:

- *Reduced Acid Reflux Symptoms*: By avoiding foods that trigger acid production and following the diet's guidelines, individuals can experience less frequent and less severe episodes of acid reflux.
- *Decreased Heartburn*: The diet helps minimize the occurrence of heartburn by reducing the likelihood of stomach acid entering the esophagus.
- *Improved Digestive Health*: Eating smaller, more frequent meals and avoiding hard-to-digest foods aids in overall digestion and can prevent the uncomfortable

fullness and bloating often associated with hiatal hernia.

- **Better Esophageal Health**: By minimizing acid reflux and irritation, the diet can help protect the esophagus from damage such as inflammation, ulcers, or scarring.
- **Enhanced Nutrient Absorption**: Proper food choices and eating habits can lead to better nutrient absorption and utilization by the body.
- **Weight Management**: Following the diet may promote weight loss or help maintain a healthy weight, which can alleviate pressure on the stomach and reduce symptoms.
- **Increased Comfort during Sleep**: Avoiding late-night meals and maintaining an upright posture after eating can lead to more restful sleep without the discomfort of night-time reflux.
- **Lifestyle Improvement**: The diet encourages overall healthier eating habits, which can have positive effects on other aspects of health beyond the management of hiatal hernia symptoms.

By adhering to these dietary principles, individuals with a hiatal hernia can often find some relief from their symptoms and may also benefit from broader positive health impacts.

Disadvantages of Hiatal Hernia Diet

While the benefits of the Hiatal Hernia diet generally outweigh the disadvantages, there are some potential drawbacks to consider:

- *Dietary Restrictions*: The diet may require cutting out certain foods and beverages that many people enjoy, such as coffee, chocolate, and spicy foods, which can be challenging for some individuals.
- *Social and Lifestyle Adjustments*: Social events and dining out can be more difficult when following a strict diet, as it can limit options and require careful planning.
- *Initial Adjustment Period*: Those new to the diet may experience an adjustment period where they need to learn what foods trigger their symptoms and how to effectively substitute ingredients in meals.
- *Possible Nutrient Deficiencies*: Restrictive diets can sometimes lead to nutrient deficiencies if not properly managed, so individuals may need to be mindful of getting a balanced intake of vitamins and minerals.
- *Additional Effort and Time*: Planning meals, reading labels, and preparing food at home can require extra effort and time, which may be inconvenient for some individuals with busy lifestyles.

- *Psychological Impact*: Constantly managing a diet can be mentally taxing and may affect one's relationship with food, potentially leading to stress or anxiety.

Despite these disadvantages, the benefits of the Hiatal Hernia diet often outweigh these challenges for those who suffer from hiatal hernia symptoms. The reduction in acid reflux, heartburn, and other uncomfortable symptoms can significantly improve quality of life.

Additionally, adopting healthier eating habits can have positive effects that extend beyond the management of hiatal hernia, contributing to overall well-being and long-term health.

Foods to Eat

If you're managing a Hiatal Hernia, your diet should focus on foods that are easy to digest and that can help minimize symptoms like acid reflux. Here's a list of foods that are generally recommended:

- *Fruits and Vegetables*: Opt for non-citrus fruits like apples, pears, bananas, melons, and berries. For vegetables, choose leafy greens, carrots, peas, green beans, and squash. These are less likely to cause reflux.

- *Lean Proteins*: Incorporate lean meats such as turkey, chicken, and fish. Eggs and tofu are also good protein sources that are gentle on the stomach.
- *Whole Grains*: Foods like oatmeal, brown rice, quinoa, and whole-grain bread and pasta provide fiber, which is important for gastrointestinal health.
- *Healthy Fats*: Include moderate amounts of healthy fats, such as avocados, nuts, seeds, and olive oil, which are essential for overall health.
- *Non-Fat or Low-Fat Dairy*: Choose products like skim milk, low-fat yogurt, and cottage cheese to get your calcium without a high-fat content that could trigger reflux.
- *Herbal Teas*: Non-caffeinated herbal teas like chamomile or ginger tea can be soothing to the stomach.

It's also important to avoid or limit foods that may exacerbate symptoms, such as high-fat foods, spicy foods, chocolate, caffeine, alcohol, carbonated beverages, and acidic foods like tomatoes and citrus fruits. Eating smaller, more frequent meals rather than large ones and avoiding eating right before bedtime can also help manage Hiatal Hernia symptoms.

Foods to Avoid

When managing a Hiatal Hernia, certain foods are known to exacerbate symptoms such as acid reflux and are best avoided or limited. Here are some types of foods and beverages that you might consider avoiding:

- *Citrus Fruits*: Oranges, grapefruits, lemons, and limes can trigger acid reflux due to their acidity.
- *Tomatoes*: As with citrus, the natural acidity in tomatoes and tomato-based products can prompt reflux symptoms.
- *Spicy Foods*: Ingredients like chili peppers and hot sauces can irritate the esophagus and stomach lining.
- *High-Fat Foods*: Fatty cuts of meat, fried foods, butter, and high-fat desserts can slow down digestion and increase the likelihood of reflux.
- *Chocolate*: It contains methylxanthine, which can relax the muscle that controls the esophageal sphincter, leading to reflux.
- *Onions and Garlic*: These can be triggers for some individuals, causing discomfort and reflux.
- *Caffeinated Beverages*: Coffee, tea, and energy drinks can aggravate an already sensitive digestive system.
- *Alcoholic Beverages*: Alcohol can relax the lower esophageal sphincter, exacerbating reflux symptoms.
- *Carbonated Drinks*: Soda and other carbonated beverages can bloat the stomach, increasing pressure and potentially worsening Hiatal Hernia symptoms.
- *Mint*: Peppermint and spearmint can relax the lower esophageal sphincter, leading to acid reflux.

- *Processed Foods*: High in salt, fat, and additives, these can trigger or worsen symptoms.

Individual responses to these foods can vary, so it's important to monitor your symptoms and determine which specific foods cause issues for you. Adjusting your diet based on your personal tolerance levels will help in managing the condition effectively.

Meal Planning and Eating Habits

The Importance of Meal Timing and Frequency

Consistency in meal timing can help stabilize the body's internal clock, aiding digestion. Spacing out meals evenly throughout the day ensures that the stomach is not too full, which can increase pressure on the hiatal hernia:

- *Regular Meal Times*: Aim to eat at the same times every day to regulate digestive processes.
- *Smaller, Frequent Meals*: Instead of three large meals, consider having 4-6 smaller meals to prevent the stomach from becoming overly full and putting pressure on the hernia.

Tips for Portion Control to Avoid Overeating

Controlling how much you eat at each sitting can significantly impact hiatal hernia symptoms:

- *Use Smaller Plates*: This can naturally encourage smaller portions without feeling deprived.
- *Listen to Your Body*: Eat slowly and pay attention to your body's signals of satiety to avoid overeating.
- *Don't Eat from the Package*: Serve snacks on plates instead of eating from the package to control quantity.

The Significance of Eating Posture and Its Effects on Symptoms

How you sit or stand while eating, and immediately after, can influence hiatal hernia discomfort:

- *Sit Upright*: When eating, sit up straight. Slouching or lying down can increase the likelihood of acid reflux.
- *Stay Upright After Meals*: Try to stay upright for at least an hour after eating; gravity will help keep stomach contents down.

Suggestions for Gentle and Effective Food Preparation Techniques

The way food is prepared can alter its potential to affect hiatal hernia symptoms:

- *Gentle Cooking Methods*: Baking, poaching, steaming, and grilling are preferable to frying or other methods that introduce a lot of fat.
- *Avoid Trigger Ingredients*: When seasoning food, use herbs that are less likely to cause acid reflux, such as

basil, thyme, and oregano, rather than chili powder or garlic.

Incorporating these meal planning and eating habits into your daily routine can play a crucial role in managing hiatal hernia symptoms. Adjust these suggestions to fit personal preferences and symptom responses for the best results.

Sample Recipes

Squash and Spinach Medley

Ingredients:

- 1 butternut squash, deseeded and sliced lengthwise
- 1 handful fresh baby spinach
- 2 tbsp. oil
- 1/4 tsp. sea salt
- 1-1/2 cups bone broth
- 1/2 tsp. Braggs Liquid Aminos
- 1 beet, sliced
- 2 tbsp. cashew yogurt

Instructions:

1. Preheat the oven to 425°F. Line a baking sheet with foil.
2. Brush 2 teaspoons of oil onto each half of the butternut squash. Season with salt.
3. Place each half on the baking sheet, flesh side down.
4. Place inside the oven and bake for 30 minutes until the flesh is soft.
5. Scoop the flesh out and place it on a high-speed blender. Add in baby spinach and bone broth. Puree until a smooth consistency is achieved.
6. Season with Braggs liquid aminos.
7. Garnish with beets and yogurt.
8. Serve and enjoy.

Fresh Asparagus Salad

Ingredients:

- 1/3 cup of hazelnuts
- 4 cups arugula
- 1 tsp. ground pepper
- 4 tsp. lemon juice
- 2 tbsp. sea salt
- virgin olive oil
- 2 lbs. asparagus

Instructions:

1. Preheat the oven to 400°F.
2. Place hazelnuts on a baking tray with parchment paper. Place in the oven for 7 minutes.
3. Transfer hazelnuts to a plate. Optionally, to remove the skins, wrap the nuts in a towel and rub them vigorously.
4. Chop hazelnuts coarsely.
5. Remove the hard ends of the asparagus.
6. Place the stalks on the baking sheet you've used for the hazelnuts. Sprinkle 1 tbsp. olive oil and 1/2 tsp. of salt.
7. Bake for 8 minutes.
8. In a mixing bowl, combine pepper, salt, olive oil, and lemon juice. Mix well.

9. Place arugula in a medium bowl. Drizzle ½ of the dressing over the veggies. Toss until everything is well coated.

10. Place arugula onto a platter.

11. Arrange asparagus on top. Sprinkle peeled hazelnuts on top.

Macrobiotic Bowl Medley

Ingredients:

- 1/2 cup brown rice
- 3 cup chard, roughly chopped
- 1 cup squash, diced
- 1 cup broccoli florets
- 1 cup black beans, thoroughly rinsed and drained
- 1 oz. kombu
- 1/2 cup sauerkraut, chopped

Sauce:

- 2 tbsp. sesame tahini
- 2 tbsp. sodium tamari
- 1 clove garlic
- 1 tbsp. ginger
- 1 lime, juiced

Instructions:

1. Boil 1 cup of water.
2. Add rice and allow it to boil. Cover and reduce heat and simmer for 40 minutes.
3. Remove from heat and allow to sit covered for another 10 minutes, then fluff with a fork.
4. Place beans in a pot with a kombu. Cover with water, and bring to a boil.

5. Reduce heat and simmer for 15-20 minutes. Drain and rinse after.

6. Place a steamer basket in a pot with water and bring to a boil.

7. Add broccoli, cover, and steam for 4-5 minutes then remove, keeping water in the pot.

8. Add squash, cover, and steam for 4-5 minutes then remove, keeping water in the pot.

9. Add chard, cover, and steam for 3-4 minutes, then remove.

10. Mix all the ingredients of the sauce.

11. Serve everything on a plate and enjoy!

Sun Crust Turkey Cuts

Ingredients:

- 2 turkey breasts, cut into 1/4-inch thick slices
- 1-1/2 cups sunflower seeds
- 1/4 tsp. ground cumin
- 2 tbsp. chopped parsley
- 1/4 tsp. paprika
- 1/4 tsp. cayenne pepper
- 1/4 tsp. black pepper
- 1/3 cup whole wheat flour
- 3 egg whites

Instructions:

1. Preheat the oven to around 395 °F.
2. Mix the parsley, paprika, cumin, cayenne, sunflower seeds, and pepper in a processor.
3. Prepare the whites and flour in a separate container each.
4. Coat each breast part with the mixtures separately. Start with the flour mixture, followed by the whites, and then the processed mixture.
5. After coating all the breasts, prepare the pan.

6. Bake the breasts for approximately 12 minutes in the oven.
7. Flip each side and resume baking for another 12 minutes.
8. Serve hot.

Arugula and Mushroom Salad

Ingredients:

- 5 oz. arugula washed
- 1 lb. fresh mushrooms
- 1/4 tsp. shoyu
- 1/2 red onion
- 1 tbsp. olive oil
- 1 tbsp. mirin

For tofu cheese:

- 1/8 cup umeboshi vinegar
- 1/2 firm tofu

Instructions:

1. In a bowl, add the rinsed tofu. Crumble and pour in vinegar.
2. In a separate bowl add shoyu, red onions, salt, olive oil, and mirin. 3. Mix to combine.
3. Add in the arugula and toss to combine with the dressing.
4. Serve and enjoy.

Cauliflower and Mushroom Bake

Ingredients:

- 3 cups cauliflower florets
- 1 cup fresh mushroom, chopped
- 1/2 cup red onion, chopped
- 1/3 cup green onion, chopped
- 2 garlic cloves, finely chopped
- 2 tsp. apple cider vinegar
- 2 tsp. lemon juice
- 1/2 tsp. salt
- 1/4 tsp. pepper
- 1 tbsp. olive oil

Instructions:

1. Preheat the oven to 350°F. Lightly grease a baking pan.
2. Combine red onion, cauliflower, olive oil, garlic, mushroom, apple cider vinegar, lemon juice, salt, and pepper in a bowl. Mix well.
3. Pour the mixture into the greased baking pan.
4. Place inside the oven and bake for 45 minutes. Stir.
5. When vegetables are golden brown and tender, remove from the oven.
6. Garnish with green onions. Serve and enjoy.

Fruit Salad with Zesty Vinaigrette

Ingredients:

- 3 mangoes, medium-sized, peeled and sliced thinly
- 3 ripe avocados, medium-sized, peeled and thinly sliced
- 1 cup blackberries, fresh
- 1 cup raspberries, fresh
- 1/4 cup mint, fresh and minced
- 1/4 cup almonds, toasted and sliced

For the dressing:

- 1 tsp. grated tangerine or orange peel
- 1/2 cup olive oil
- 1/2 tsp. salt
- 1/4 cup tangerine or orange juice
- 1/4 tsp. freshly ground pepper
- 2 tbsp. balsamic vinegar

Instructions:

1. Combine all the fruits on a serving plate.
2. Sprinkle the salad with mint and almonds.
3. Whisk together all the dressing ingredients in a smaller bowl.
4. Drizzle the dressing over the salad.
5. Consume after serving.

Orange-Walnut Salad

Ingredients:

- 2 cups romaine lettuce, chopped coarsely
- 1 cucumber, peeled and deseeded, quartered lengthwise and chopped
- 1 cup arugula
- 2 navel oranges, peeled and chopped
- 1/4 cup red onion, sliced thinly
- 1 tbsp. walnut oil
- 2 tbsp. walnuts, chopped
- 1 tbsp. red wine vinegar
- 2 oz. blue cheese, gluten-free

Instructions:

1. In a salad bowl, carefully place the ingredients into layers.
2. Sprinkle it with walnut oil and vinegar and toss.
3. With your hands, crumble blue cheese on top.
4. Serve immediately and enjoy.

Korean-Style Cauliflower

Ingredients:

- 1 cauliflower, cut into small florets
- 1 tbsp. cornstarch
- pepper
- baking soda

For the batter:

- 1 cup all-purpose flour
- 1/2 cup cornstarch
- 2 tsp. baking powder
- 1 tbsp. garlic powder
- 1 cup water

For the sauce:

- 1-1/2 tbsp Korean chili sauce
- 4 tbsp. low-sodium soy sauce
- 3 tbsp. honey
- 1 tsp. sesame oil
- 1/2 tsp. grated ginger
- 1/2 tsp. minced garlic
- 1/4 tsp. rice vinegar

For the garnish:

- lime zest
- sesame seeds

- lime wedges
- ranch dressing
- green onions

Instructions:

1. In a small bowl, add a tablespoon of cornstarch with baking powder and pepper.
2. Put the cauliflower florets on a flat surface and sprinkle the cornstarch mixture over it.
3. In a large bowl, add the ingredients for the batter and whisk them together. While whisking, add water to create a thick batter.
4. Dip the cauliflower florets into the batter and place the florets on a wire rack to let the excess batter drip off.
5. Lightly coat the air fryer basket with cooking spray. Put the florets into the basket in a single layer.
6. Cook florets for 12 minutes at 350°F. Let the florets become golden brown. Repeat the process with other florets.
7. Put all the sauce ingredients in a saucepan. Bring the mixture to a simmer. Once it becomes thick, remove it from heat.
8. Put the cooked cauliflower in a large bowl. Pour the sauce over the florets and toss to coat.
9. Garnish the florets as desired.
10. Serve it with ranch dressing.

Blackberry Cobbler

Ingredients:

- 2 tbsp. organic coconut oil, with an additional amount for greasing
- 1/4 cup arrowroot flour
- 12 oz. blackberries
- 1/4 cup raw honey
- 3 tbsp. water
- 1/4 tsp. salt
- 1-1/4 tsp. lemon juice
- 3/4 tsp. baking soda
- 1/4 cup coconut flour

Instructions:

1. Preheat the oven to 300°F.
2. Use coconut oil to grease an 8×8 baking dish.
3. Place blackberries at the bottom of the pan, ensuring that they are placed evenly.
4. Place the remaining ingredients in a food processor. Pulse at medium speed until thoroughly combined and then spread over blackberries.
5. Bake for 35 to 40 minutes or until the top turns golden brown.
6. Serve and enjoy.

Low-Cholesterol Apple-Cinnamon Granola Breakfast

Ingredients:

- 3 cups regular oats
- 2 tbsp. butter
- 1 cup whole-grain oat cereal
- 1/3 cup applesauce
- 1/3 cup oat bran
- 1/4 cup honey
- 1/3 cup walnuts, finely chopped
- 2 tbsp. brown sugar
- 2 tsp. ground cinnamon
- 1 cup dried apple, finely chopped
- 1/4 tsp. ground cardamom

Instructions:

1. Preheat the oven until it reaches the temperature of 250°F.
2. Combine regular oats, oat cereal, oat bran, walnuts, cinnamon, and cardamom in a large bowl.
3. Stir well to combine the ingredients thoroughly.
4. Melt two tablespoons of butter in a saucepan over medium heat.
5. Add honey, brown sugar, and 1/3 cup of applesauce into the heated saucepan. Boil.

6. Cook the mixture for a minute. Pour the applesauce mixture on top of the oat mixture while stirring well to coat.
7. Spread the resulting mixture in a jelly roll pan.
8. Coat the jelly roll pan with cooking spray.
9. Bake the mixture at 250°F for 90 minutes while stirring frequently every 30 minutes. Let it cool.
10. Stir finely chopped apples into the granola. Store them in an airtight container.

Grapefruit and Spinach Smoothie

Ingredients:

- 1 grapefruit
- 1 cup coconut milk
- 1 cup spinach
- a pinch of Stevia to sweeten

Instructions:

1. Put all the ingredients in the blender.
2. Blend well.
3. Serve and enjoy.

Chicken Rice Noodles

Ingredients:

- 1 cup rice, uncooked
- 1 tbsp. oil, preferably coconut or vegetable
- 1-1/2 cups medium noodles
- 3 cups chicken stock
- salt
- pepper

Instructions:

1. Pour oil into a pot. Once hot, put in brown rice.
2. Add in noodles and the chicken stock. Season with salt and pepper.
3. Bring the mixture to a boil. Once boiling, reduce the heat. Cook for 20 minutes without cover, until the rice and noodles are tender and ready to eat.
4. Serve and enjoy.

Baked Turkey Wings

Ingredients:

- 4 pcs. or about 5 lbs. whole turkey wings
- 1 tbsp. olive oil
- salt
- pepper
- 1 tsp. paprika

Instructions:

1. Preheat the oven to 375°F.
2. Use foil to line a baking pan.
3. Remove the wing tips and fat. Separate from the drumette.
4. Place on the rack and drizzle with olive oil.
5. Season with pepper and salt.
6. Roast turkey wings until cooked.
7. Sprinkle paprika over the wings upon serving.

Spinach, Feta, and Tomato Omelet

Ingredients:

- cooking spray
- 1/4 cup Roma tomatoes, chopped
- 3/4 cup Egg Beaters Liquid Egg Whites
- 2 tbsp. fat-reduced feta cheese, crumbled
- 1/8 tsp. ground black pepper
- 1/4 cup baby spinach leaves, chopped

Instructions:

1. Spray small amounts of cooking spray in a nonstick skillet. Heat over medium heat.
2. Cook the Egg Beaters in the skillet, and season with pepper. Cook for 2 minutes.
3. Lift the edges to cook the other side of the egg. Cook for 3 more minutes.
4. Top half of the omelet with tomatoes, spinach, and feta cheese. Fold the other half of the omelet over the filling.
5. Serve.

Oatmeal with Sliced Bananas

Ingredients:

- 1/2 cup rolled oats
- 1 cup almond milk or water
- 1 ripe banana, sliced
- Pinch of cinnamon (optional)

Instructions:

1. Combine the rolled oats and almond milk (or water) in a medium-sized saucepan.
2. Place the saucepan over medium heat and bring the mixture to a simmer.
3. Cook for about 5 to 7 minutes, stirring occasionally, until the oats are fully cooked and have absorbed most of the liquid.
4. Remove the pan from heat and let the oatmeal sit for 1 minute to thicken further.
5. Pour the oatmeal into a serving bowl.
6. Top the oatmeal with the sliced banana and add a pinch of cinnamon if desired.
7. Serve warm and enjoy a nutritious start to your day.

Creamy Carrot Soup

Ingredients:

- 1 lb carrots, peeled and chopped
- 1 medium onion, chopped
- 4 cups of reduced-sodium vegetable stock
- 1/4 cup low-fat Greek yogurt (or dairy-free alternative)
- 1 tablespoon olive oil
- Salt to taste
- Black pepper to taste
- Fresh herbs for garnish (parsley, dill, or chives work well)

Instructions:

1. Heat the olive oil in a large pot over medium heat.
2. Add the chopped onions to the pot and sauté until they become translucent and slightly golden, around 5 minutes.
3. Add the chopped carrots to the pot, stirring them in with the onions. Cook for another 5 minutes until the carrots start to soften.
4. Pour the low-sodium vegetable broth into the pot with the onions and carrots.
5. Bring to a boil, then reduce to a simmer. Cover and let cook for about 20-25 minutes or until the carrots are very tender.

6. Once the carrots are soft, remove the pot from heat. Using an immersion blender, blend the soup directly in the pot until smooth.

7. If you don't have an immersion blender, carefully transfer the soup in batches to a blender and blend until smooth. Be sure to allow steam to escape when blending hot liquids.

8. Return the blended soup to the pot if using a stand blender.

9. Over low heat, stir in the Greek yogurt until fully integrated into the soup. Season with salt and black pepper to taste. Be gentle with the heat to prevent the yogurt from curdling.

10. Serve the soup warm, garnished with a dollop of Greek yogurt and fresh herbs.

Conclusion

Congratulations on reaching the end of this comprehensive guide on managing a hiatal hernia through diet! By now, you've equipped yourself with valuable knowledge that empowers you to take charge of your health and mitigate the discomfort associated with this condition. Remember, the journey towards better health is both rewarding and challenging, but by adopting the dietary strategies discussed, you're already making significant strides toward relief and well-being.

Understanding the impact of a hiatal hernia on your body is the first step in conquering its symptoms. You've learned that the types of food you eat, the manner in which you consume them, and even the way you structure your meals throughout the day can profoundly influence the severity of your symptoms. By focusing on a balanced diet rich in fiber, and low in acidic and fatty foods, and by eating smaller, more frequent meals, you are setting the stage for a healthier digestive system.

Remember, the power to alleviate discomfort lies in your hands. Making simple yet effective changes like elevating your head while sleeping, avoiding eating right before bedtime, and maintaining a healthy weight can have a positive impact on your symptoms. These lifestyle adjustments, although they may seem small, contribute to reducing the pressure on your stomach and can prevent the backflow of stomach acid into the esophagus.

The value of staying hydrated cannot be overstated. Drinking plenty of water throughout the day aids digestion and helps maintain the balance of bodily fluids. However, be mindful of when you drink – consuming liquids in between meals as opposed to during can help minimize the risk of acid reflux.

As you move forward, keep in mind that moderation is key. While it's important to indulge occasionally, being conscious of portion sizes and the nature of your indulgences will help you maintain control over your hiatal hernia symptoms. Equally crucial is the need to listen to your body. Everyone's experience with hiatal hernia is unique, and what works for one person may not work for another. Pay attention to how your body reacts to different foods and adjust your diet accordingly.

Stress management also plays an integral role in controlling hiatal hernia symptoms. Incorporating stress-reduction techniques such as deep breathing exercises, meditation, or yoga into your routine can lead to an overall better quality of life and can potentially lessen the frequency and intensity of your symptoms.

As you embark on this dietary journey, remember to consult with healthcare professionals regularly. They can provide personalized advice and ensure that your diet complements any medical treatments you may be undergoing. Their guidance is invaluable as you navigate through the diverse dietary choices available to you.

Furthermore, consider keeping a food diary. Documenting what you eat, the time of your meals, and any symptoms you experience can offer insights into which foods and habits trigger your symptoms. This practice can lead to a more tailored and effective dietary plan that specifically addresses your individual needs.

In embracing these dietary changes, you're not just managing your hiatal hernia; you're enhancing your overall health. A balanced diet, coupled with a mindful approach to eating, can lead to improved energy levels, stronger immunity, and a more vibrant sense of well-being.

Let this guide serve as a starting point for a lifelong commitment to healthful living. With every meal, you have the opportunity to nourish your body and soothe your symptoms. Embrace the challenge with optimism, and allow each day to be a step towards feeling your best. Your dedication to managing your hiatal hernia through diet illustrates your commitment to self-care, and that alone is a significant accomplishment.

Remember, the path to managing a hiatal hernia is a gradual one, marked by persistence and adaptability. Stay encouraged, continue to educate yourself, and reach out to support groups or online communities if you need encouragement or ideas. You're not alone on this journey, and sharing experiences can be both comforting and informative.

In closing, give yourself a pat on the back for completing this guide and taking control of your health. By implementing the strategies you've learned, you're on your way to minimizing the impact of hiatal hernia on your life. Keep pushing forward with positivity, and don't let setbacks discourage you. Each day presents a new chance to live better, feel better, and enjoy your meals with contentment and confidence. Here's to your health and a brighter, symptom-free future!

FAQ

What is a hiatal hernia, and how does diet affect it?

A hiatal hernia arises when a segment of the stomach advances upwards, penetrating through the diaphragm. Your diet can significantly impact symptoms by either exacerbating or alleviating them. Certain foods can increase stomach acid and cause reflux, while others can help maintain a healthy digestive system, reducing symptoms.

Which foods should I avoid if I have a hiatal hernia?

It's recommended to avoid foods that are acidic, spicy, fatty, or fried as these can trigger heartburn and reflux symptoms. Citrus fruits, chocolate, caffeine, alcohol, onions, peppermint, and carbonated beverages are common culprits that you might consider limiting or avoiding.

Are there any specific foods that can help manage hiatal hernia symptoms?

Yes, foods that are high in fiber such as whole grains, vegetables, and fruits (non-citrus) can be beneficial, as they aid digestion and prevent constipation, which can put additional pressure on the hernia. Lean proteins and nonfat or low-fat dairy products are also advisable.

How important are meal timing and size for managing a hiatal hernia?

Meal timing and size are crucial. Eating smaller, more frequent meals instead of large ones can prevent the stomach from becoming too full, which reduces pressure on the diaphragm. Avoiding meals right before lying down or going to bed can also help minimize reflux.

Can lifestyle changes complement the dietary management of a hiatal hernia?

Absolutely. Lifestyle changes such as maintaining a healthy weight, quitting smoking, and wearing loose-fitting clothes can greatly complement dietary efforts. Additionally, elevating the head of your bed can prevent acid from flowing back into the esophagus during sleep.

Is it necessary to follow a strict diet forever if I have a hiatal hernia?

Not necessarily. The diet for managing a hiatal hernia is more about making informed choices rather than strict avoidance. Over time, you may learn what triggers your symptoms and will be able to make adjustments that suit your tolerance levels. However, consistent healthy eating habits are beneficial for overall well-being.

Should I consult a doctor or dietitian regarding my hiatal hernia diet?

Yes, consulting with a healthcare professional is always a wise decision. They can provide tailored advice that takes into account your health history and current medications. A dietitian can also help develop a meal plan that meets your nutritional needs while managing symptoms.

References and Helpful Links

Pihma-Sydney. (2023, February 17). Acupuncture for Stress Relief - PIHMA College & Clinic. PIHMA College & Clinic. https://www.pihma.edu/acupuncture-for-stress-relief/

Gastroenterology, S. (2021, April 28). Foods to eat and avoid for hiatal hernia | SMILES. Smiles Gastroenterology. https://gastroenterology.smileshospitals.com/foods-to-eat-and-avoid-for-hiatal-hernia/

Hiatal hernia. (a.n.d.). Cleveland Clinic. Retrieved August 26, 2022, from https://my.clevelandclinic.org/health/diseases/8098-hiatal-hernia. - Google Search. (n.d.). https://www.google.com/search?

Sfara, A., & Dumitraşcu, D. L. (2019). The management of hiatal hernia: an update on diagnosis and treatment. Medicine and Pharmacy Reports. https://doi.org/10.15386/mpr-1323

Phillips, Q. (2023, January 4). What is a hiatal hernia? Symptoms, causes, diagnosis, treatment, and prevention. EverydayHealth.com. https://www.everydayhealth.com/hiatal-hernia/guide/

Christiansen, S. (2023, September 19). What to eat when you have a hiatal hernia. Verywell Health. https://www.verywellhealth.com/hiatal-hernia-diet-4773046

Marks, H. (2011, February 1). Hiatal hernia diet tips. WebMD. https://www.webmd.com/digestive-disorders/hiatal-hernia-diet-tips

Hiatal hernia symptoms + 5 Hiatal hernia natural remedies - Dr. Axe. (2023, February 18). Dr. Axe. https://draxe.com/health/hiatal-hernia/

Made in the USA
Coppell, TX
30 November 2024

41453106R00046